Halitosis: Bad Breath Causes and Natural Treatment Solutions

Written By: Alyson Rodgers

Disclaimer

Published by:
Alyson Rodgers and Random Technologies
4409 HOFFNER AVENUE, SUITE 347
Belle Isle, FL 32812

TABLE OF CONTENTS

Introduction

Have you ever been talking to someone, having a good conversation, only to notice their nose cringe – and realizing it's because of your breath? Or maybe your friends make a regular habit of passing you the mints at break.

We've all been there. At one time or another, everyone struggles with bad breath in their lifetime. Maybe you forgot to brush your teeth, maybe you had the garlic onion sandwich for lunch, or maybe, like millions of others throughout the world, you are experiencing a struggle with halitosis (bad breath).

If you're wondering if you may have a problem with halitosis, but aren't sure how to assess it yourself, feel free to seek out the opinion of a trusted friend or loved one. Let them know what you're worrying about, make it easy for them to be honest, because if you do – it's far from the end of the world.

Symptoms of bad breath
- Bad taste in your mouth
- Slight layer of film on your tongue
- You are always offered mints, even when others are not
- People sometimes noticeably back away from you when you're talking to them

No matter what the cause is that day, having bad

breath doesn't make any one feel good. It's something we should all learn to deal with, whether we're battling bad breath today or just know it comes up from time to time. Fear not, halitosis is completely treatable!

The key is to understand that you are not alone in this battle! People often suffer in silence with bad breath, fearing embarrassment, or thinking that there's nothing that can be done. Nothing could be further from the truth. By facing up to the fact that you have bad breath, you enable yourself to move forward with *treating* that bad breath – to make this problem a thing of the past before you know it.

This guide will overviews not just what bad breath is and what its underlying causes are, but also a myriad of treatment options to leave you feeling better and fresher on a regular basis. We'll help you understand what the root of the issue is, and how to deal with it, to ensure your long term success.

Halitosis – Everything You Need to Know

What are we talking About Here?
This guide is looking into halitosis (chronically bad breath). This condition is one that involves chronically having an issue with foul smelling breath, and can be treated – but not before we get over the issues we build up surrounding it.

Persistent Condition

It should be noted that although this is a common problem, this is not the same issue as the occasional bout of "morning breath". Morning breath is a culturally accepted phenomenon, but unless its occurring with increased frequency, should not be of concern.

Bad breath comes in two varieties, transient and chronic. Transient bad breath is temporary, coming and going due to any number of factors, and generally battle-able with an increased emphasis on oral hygiene and watching what you eat. Chronic bad breath however, is what's known as halitosis.

Halitosis is a condition. A condition that seems to ignore the hygienic levels of its user, in favor of surviving despite your use of toothpaste. This is what we're talking about here, this is what can be treated, but will not go away without treatment.

People who suffer from halitosis often worry they will be thought of as dirty, or having poor hygiene habits, but bad breath often ignores even the best hygiene habits. This does not mean that you should give up on oral hygiene though, proper brushing and flossing are absolutely essential as a foundation to your battle with bad breath.

The Problem of Bad Breath?

You often aren't aware that bad breath is an issue *until* someone else around you reacts! This is the root of the embarrassment that all too often attacks victims of halitosis.

No one wants to speak up and admit that it's their breath that stinks, or knows how to handle a friend constantly stepping backwards to avoid smelling them, but the truth is that this is a problem that almost everyone has to face. In fact, bad breath is something we don't even like to admit to a medical professional – making it all the more difficult to get help!

This is the other issue, bad breath effects everyone. Halitosis is not restricted by gender, by income, by age, or even by culture. It can effect any one, and it likely will.

The Many Potential Causes of Bad Breath

There are several potential causes of bad breath, let's look at the list and then consider how you can best isolate your particular cause.

The Causes of Bad Breath

The cause of halitosis can be difficult to isolate. Bad breath can be caused from nearly anything, from improper brushing, to the garlic sandwich you ate. In fact, did you know that bad breath can even be your body's away of warning you that something else is going wrong? Bad breath has been associated with the presence of infection, kidney and liver issues, diabetes, bronchitis, and even stomach issues.

It's even more important to understand that it can have multiple underlying causes, not just one thing or another.

So how can we begin to understand the causes of bad breath? Let's consider the smell itself. Bad breath is a reflection of a foul smell, this smell can be traced to one of five locations within the mouth – each with their own causes and potential reasons for existing, but locations to work with nonetheless.

What are these five locations?
- Chronic habits, such as smoking
- The posterior dorsum on the tongue
- Dentures – Dentures can retain a terrible odor, particularly if stored improperly
- Periodontal (dental floss or crevicular fluid in the periodontal sectors of the mouth)
- Nasal odor can often appear to be a bad breath issue, but really be an issue within the nasal cavity.

Each of these areas from within the mouth and body are dream hideaways for the bacteria that can lead to the oh so irritating bad breath we're talking about here. Interestingly, it's important to keep hydrated when trying to deal with bad breath, as an excessively dry mouth is one of the biggest ways to set the stage for the growth of foul smelling bacteria.

It is important to note that keeping your mouth from being dry may or may not be within your control. For example, medications often naturally dry out the mouth, and this has been known to lead to halitosis. This guide focuses on the factors you can control, and ways of minimizing the impact of the factors that you can't.

A Non-Comprehensive List:
- Alcohol
- Allergies
- Bacterias
- Stomach problems
- Gum disease
- Dialysis
- Diet
- Dehydration
- Simple leftover food
- Oral infections, conditions, and cancers
- Malnutrition
- Menstruation
- A persistently dry mouth (often referred to as Xerostomia)

- Damage to liver or kidneys (particularly cirrhosis in the liver)
- An excessively dry mouth
- Poor oral hygiene habits
- Sinus infections
- Tonsil infections
- Respiratory infections
- Renal failure
- Uremia
- Fevers
- Smoking (nicotine and tobacco)
- Spicy foods
- Systematic diseases and disorders

Bacteria as a Cause of Bad Breath

Typically, halitosis has been linked to an excess of foul smelling bacteria, and it is by dealing with those bacteria that we will deal with your halitosis.

There are two types of bacteria, aerobes (oxygen dependent) and anaerobes (oxygen independent), that help your body to function. Aerobes are the primary culprit in halitosis, in that they are also responsible for other bodily stimulation – such as stimulation of sulfur. Sulfuric compounds are the foul smell, or bad taste, that bad breath frequently leaves in our mouths.

Now, bacteria naturally occurs within your body. This is not bad, in fact, if you didn't have these types of bacteria it would be bad for you, but too much or too little creates an imbalance that can lead to problems like halitosis. If you have too many aerobes for example, your body produces excess amounts of the smelly VSCs (Sulfuric substances within the body).

Food
Now that you have an understanding of aerobes and anaerobes, you may be wondering if there is anything dietary you do to increase a potential imbalance. The answer is a resounding yes! Food has differing effects on the body, and thus on the body's stimulation of bacteria, and storage of bacteria for that matter.

Recall that halitosis thrives in excessively dry environments, and consider that some foods dry your mouth. There are certainly things you can do when considering your diet to combat potentially bad breath.

So what can you do?

Consider what the food you are eating is doing to your body. There are four primary classifications of food – protein foods, acidic foods, sugars, and drying. As you can imagine, each category has its own effects on your body.

It should be noted that none of these foods can (or should) be completely avoided for their bad breath inducing properties, it's merely good to make yourself aware of these properties so you can combat them where possible, and consume in moderation elsewhere.

Proteins
Examples: -Beef -Dairy -Fish
Foods that are high in protein are often low in carbohydrates. This forces the body to rely on fat stores for energy, and releases foul smelling ketones throughout your body. What's the solution? If you have persistently bad breath, consume these foods in lower doses where possible.

Acidic Foods
Examples: Juice (orange, pineapple, tomato), Decaf coffee

This and sugar are foods that have the potential to imbalance your bacteria, leading to halitosis. This doesn't mean you can't drink them, just drink in moderation.

Sugars
The examples seem evident, and the reality is clear, sugar is bad for you. In the case of bad breath, sugar has been implicated for its decaying properties, in creating issues that set the stage for halitosis.

Drying Foods
Examples: -Alcohol -Nicotine -Tobacco

Drying foods, as the name suggests, dry out the mouth (making it easier for bacteria to thrive). Make sure you are working extra hard to keep yourself hydrated when ingesting these foods, if you do not you are setting the stage for VSCs to thrive and halitosis to remain.

The final word on how diet effects your breath is related to your oral hygiene habits. Food particles of any kind that remain within the mouth are breeding grounds for bacteria, and can go bad and cause their own stench. It is for this reason that it is absolutely critical that you brush, and floss, at least once a day (preferably after each meal).

Periodontal Disease (Gum Disease)
Symptoms of gum disease
- Frequent bleeding in the gums
- Gum separation from teeth or teeth separating
- Swelling or tenderness in the gums
- Constant bad taste within the mouth
- Bad breath

A good rule of thumb is that if your breath is particularly potent just after flossing, you likely have gum disease of some kind. Research has consistently linked gum disease and bad breath, from as early as 2001. This is thought to be because the saliva in those with gum disease contains a stench that can cause bad breath, and bacterias are more attracted to infected gums.

Gum disease is an infection in your gums. This infection hides in the sulcus, the small space between your teeth and gums. Gum disease has two classifications, much like the classifications of bad breath (chronic or temporary); gingivitis and periodontitis.

Now, don't panic if you've heard you have gingivitis, this is extremely common – and can be dealt with. Even periodontitis has its treatments, the key is to identify if this is the cause of your bad breath.

Conclusion
There are many potential causes to bad breath. The first step to determining your causes is elimination, so head out to that doctor and book that dentist appointment! You need to know if your halitosis could actually be something more systematically wrong with your body, for the sake of not only your breath but also your health!

We will now look onward to specific treatments for halitosis and how they can help you.

The Worst Things You Can Do for Halitosis

When people have an issue they're embarrassed about, they often take matters into their own hands long before submitting to the hands of a professional. This is a mistake which we will discuss in the next chapter, but this chapter will overview the top 10 worst ideas for halitosis battling.

- They drink! Alcohol only serves to dry your mouth, causing further problems.

- Breath mints – they only mask the problem, and often actually are high in sugar which is terrible for your body!

- Excessive use of mouthwash

- Using the wrong kind of mouthwash – See our next chapter for the best advice on how to select your mouthwash, because using the wrong kind can actually aggravate your halitosis.

- Chewing gum – Again, only temporary, only a mask. With halitosis, the key is to treat the problem, not hide it.

- Mint chew tobacco – This is actually associated with the loss of bone and receding gums, and can lead to far more serious conditions – on top of not helping with halitosis.

- Trying to use cleansers within the mouth – This is terribly unfortunate as it has poisonously harmful effects on the body.

- Infomercial items – Do not believe anything you see on TV. Only use products that are known to be approved of by the American Dental Association. This will ensure you are exercising at least SOME caution, but this too is not a good idea without the advice of a medical professional.

- Intestinal cleansers – Generally ineffective in the battle against halitosis

- Tongue piercings – Actually create more surface area for bacteria to hide, thus increasing issues with halitosis

Don't misunderstand me, these mistakes do not make their makers stupid in any way. These are common mistakes that unfortunately only serve to aggravate halitosis, and in many cases harm the sufferer more than they help.

Traditional Treatments for Halitosis

Treatment for halitosis comes in waves, from improving your oral hygiene habits to paying attention to your particular causes of bad breath. The first step to any effective treatment however? A visit to the family physician.

We've already discussed at length how many health problems are linked with bad breath, it is important to rule out health issues, or treat them if they are your cause. A visit to your family doctor can help assess your physical health, and thus tell you if it could be something else that's causing your halitosis.

Already been to the family doctor? Try your dentist, and make sure that they know that you've already been to the doctor. By involving medical professionals, you're able to rule out health issues and things like gum disease, narrowing down your cause of bad breath, and thus your treatment options, substantially.

What to do at the Doctors and Dentist for Bad Breath
The key to an effective battle with bad breath is involving the medical professionals, but what do you need to do to help these appointments along? There are a few things, the key being the way you prepare for the appointments themselves.

Step 1) Make sure you are clear when booking the appointment that this is about a bad breath issue

This enables your physician and dentist to be aware of what you're coming in for, ask

preliminary questions, and potentially even pull together some treatment options ahead of time.

Step 2) Prepare yourself

This means you need to avoid anything that's going to inhibit your physician or dentist from

being able to smell the problem. No alcohol, try to avoid smoking, chewing gum, candies, or

other strong smelling substances that may mask the issue. This enables your physician to tell if   it is a specific odor related to certain health issues. The following is a list of recommended

advice for the day before the appointment:

- Do not book the appointment if you have been on antibiotics within the last three weeks
- No cabbage, garlic, or onions for 2 days leading up to the appointment
- No brushing, flossing, or using mouthwash for 12 hours prior to your appointment
- No smoking or consuming of alcohol for 12 hours prior to your appointment.
- Drink only water for 5 hours leading up to the appointment itself
- Try to avoid any type of scent (candy, perfume, aftershave, etc.)

In terms of what will happen at the appointment itself, your professional will likely ask you for a history of your treatments so far and examine the area. They may recommend a starter treatment, or (if a dentist) perform a cleaning to try to eradicate the problem off the start. They may also send you on to another specialist.

The events that will likely take place at a dentist will be a little more specialized to the issue at hand. The appointment will typically begin with a smell assessment of the practitioner themselves, and possibly a halimeter reading (halimeters measure the presence of VSCs within the mouth in a parts per billion rate). They will likely follow this up with x-rays and a collection of your medical history. This is all part of a normal appointment, and should be done before other treatments are undergone by yourself.

Remember to be receptive to their advice, they are the trained professional. If the problem persists, *that* is when you look further.

Once you have eliminated health as a cause of bad breath, you can start looking into treatments that impact the other potential causes. Let's go through the dos, and do-not's, to give you an idea of how you can best help yourself overcome halitosis.

The Do's
Oral Hygiene – Your First Line of Defense

While bad breath is not necessarily caused by poor oral hygiene habits, it cannot hurt to make sure yours are at their level best when battling halitosis.

You need to be cleaning your mouth fully. This means: teeth, gums, tongue, and between your teeth (this is where flossing comes in). Note that you may need a tongue cleaner in addition to your toothbrush (some toothbrushes now come with one) and to be gentle on your gums.

The key here is consistency. You should be brushing *and* flossing your teeth every single day, for 2-3 minutes at a time. Ideally you should be brushing and flossing after every meal, but at least once a day for an appropriate amount of time.

Some people question the length of time it takes to keep their mouths clean, often spending less than a third of the required time. This is a critical error in judgement, the equivalent of skipping a third of your daily bath or a third of your night's rest – it simply leaves you ill equipped and enables halitosis to continue. Remember, bacteria has five places to hide, you want to get to each area and prevent it from continuing to fester and smell, and this effort takes time.

The reason that oral hygiene is so critical is twofold: 1) it clears the way for other treatments to kick in easier and 2) it makes it harder for bacteria to thrive in your mouth, restoring balance to the body and reducing your bad breath.

Take Care of Your Tongue
The tongue is an often neglected part of oral hygiene, but it needs to be included in a plan to battle issues with persisting bad breath. In fact, the tongue's surface is one of the areas we identified as dangerous because of its bacteria hosting abilities. (The posterior dorsum).

So how do you take care of your tongue? Take a minute and soak your toothbrush in mouthwash, then gently brush your tongue – reaching as far back as comfortably possible.

Making this a regular part of your oral hygiene routine will ensure that bacteria loses its hold on your mouth. If you continue to struggle however, this will be where you return to the dentist.

Stay Hydrated – Combat Dry Mouth
We have already talked at length about the problem of a dry mouth, it provides a breeding ground for bacteria. So how do you fight dry mouth? The simple answer is to wet it, and the best answer is to do so with water. Water not only hydrates you, it helps to clean away food and is great for both your mouth and your body. So, staying hydrated is a hugely beneficial treatment for halitosis.

See Your Dentist
Regular appointments with your dentist enable you

to stay ahead of any problems you may be having with gum disease, halitosis, abscesses, and more. Make sure you're keeping your cleaning appointments!

The Don'ts (or do carefully)
Temporary Solutions
Many people suffering from halitosis try to use mouthwashes and extra toothpaste to combat their bad breath. This can be a mistake, if one is not careful. To combat the occasional bout of morning breath, these solutions are perfect – temporary and simple. But if you are persistently struggling with halitosis, you may need to dig a little deeper to get to your causes (see the chapter above) and actually treat the problem – rather than the symptomatic bad breath.

The Do-Not's should not really be thought of as something never to indulge in, but rather to use carefully. For example, while it is true that you should not use mouthwash as your only method of combatting halitosis, it is a valid assisting aid, when carefully selected. For that reason, the Do-Not's are really more "do carefully". Don't *just* use temporary solutions to fight your issues with bad breath, be sure to look into the other lines of defences available to you.

Tools of the Trade
All of this advice is for nothing if you aren't using the right tools to improve your oral hygiene. The following are guidelines related to toothbrushes

and mouthwash.

Mouthwash Mayhem

So what's the deal with mouthwash? It can be your best friend or just another foe. You see, one of the primary ingredients in mouthwash is alcohol – a drying agent if you recall the last chapter – so it can actually hurt if not selected correctly.

But how do you select mouthwash correctly? You need to pick a mouthwash that will not just mask the bad breath but also eliminate the bacterias and VSCs responsible for the bad breath in the first place. Otherwise, unless you plan on taking mouthwash every few hours...forever... the problem is just going to return, and may even worsen depending on the type of mouthwash you are using.

Look for rinses that have chlorine dioxide, chlorhexidine gluconate, cetylpyridium chloride, and zinc to assess the quality of the mouthwash. Research has proven the value of these ingredients repeatedly, and thus you will have the greatest possible chance at eradicating your halitosis if your mouthwash makes use of them.

Picking the Right Toothbrush

Fun fact? The toothbrush form we all know and love today did not appear until the late 18th century in the United Kingdom – and not until the 19th century in the United States!

The tool of the trade, your toothbrush. Primitive references to the toothbrush have appeared as early as 1600 BC, in the form of "chewing sticks". Toothbrushes as we know them today appear to have been found in ancient Mesopotamia in as early as 3000 BC. Of course, they didn't get to use any soft bristles or floss, but they had tools like toothpicks – often crafted from flavorful woods that could be chewed.

Research has only recently (1919 and onward) implemented toothbrushes as a required standard, but thankfully in doing so have gathered necessary advice for how we should select toothbrushes today. We have the benefit of using a toothbrush instead of a chewing stick, but that doesn't mean all toothbrushes are created equal.

The American Dental Association has established the following standards for toothbrushes:
- Soft bristled (be gentle to your teeth!)
- Flexible
- Inexpensive
- Light to the touch
- Quick drying
- Efficiently designed to help your mouth get clean, and easily drying to help itself remain clean enough to continue with this job.

Alternative Treatments for Halitosis

Allopathic medicine (Western medicine) is not the only medical recourse for treating illnesses – from heartburn to halitosis – but it has been the dominant view. Many of us have grown up in places where Western medicine is presented as the only view, but this could not be further from the truth.

Before Western medicine (and indeed after), people have had great success in using naturalistic and herbal remedies for treating disease. Western medicine has been slow to recognize this truth, wanting to maintain allopathic control over the systems it presides over, but recently even the Western educational system has had to recognize that there is a range of treatment options – and allopathic medicine is only one branch of that range.

Allopathy has its place to be sure, but so does the naturalistic approach to health that considers not just medicines, but alternative treatments. It should be noted that although these treatments are classified as "alternative" they are not in any way inferior. Occasionally, the biased pharmaceutical market tries to present these treatments as "unproven" and "untested", but the truth is that these 'alternative treatments' have a considerably longer (and more successful) history than all of

Western medicine. Active research is continually being done around the globe to document these treatments, and academia in several parts of the world is ready to recognize alternative treatments' value.

In other cultures, particularly Chinese, Indian, and European, these naturalistic alternatives are often presented even before the conventional Western medicine is offered. A major component of why this has prevailed is because of the recognition in these places that alternative treatments often provide fewer side effects and the same results. This has led to the development of the term "naturopathy", a term used to describe the branch of medicine that seeks naturalistic solutions rather than allopathic solutions.

These solutions cover not just medicine, but also massage, aromatherapy, acupuncture, and many other techniques that we are more than familiar with, we just may not have thought of them as a defence for halitosis.

The bottom line is that traditional treatments are not your only lines of defence against halitosis. If mouthwash isn't working for you, or you're finding you need more than just to floss, the treatments in these pages should be regarded as viable natural options.

You should note however, you need to indulge in

these treatments only after research and careful consideration. Not using a treatment form correctly, whether allopathic or naturopathic, can result in harm coming to you. (This is often where people derive their negative reports of naturopathy – in instances where it was clearly used incorrectly). So pay attention to the notes here, and feel free to do further research where more instruction is needed.

Naturopathy exists as a holistic approach to medicine, and nobody would rush you into trying a tea before you knew its effects or how to prepare it correctly. Always choose your methods carefully.

That being said, enjoy the following list of naturalistic alternatives to allopathic medicine for halitosis! (Say that ten times fast!)

Avocado
Avocados have become known for their ability to help purify your system, they act as a general cleanser of bacterias and remaining food particles.

Bicarbonate Soda
More commonly known as baking soda, baking soda is an extremely common household ingredient that can be used as an alternate toothpaste – or a toothpaste companion if the taste becomes an issue. PLEASE remember to rinse all of the baking soda out of your mouth afterwards, or you may be left with a nastier taste than when you started with.

Cranberries
Cranberries create an environment that makes it more difficult for bacteria (or plaque for that matter) to form and remain within your mouth. This is a great way to contribute to your oral hygiene!

Guava
Guava is a fruit that helps the health of your gums, and can even stop bleeding if you chew on its leaves for a few minutes! This fruit is a wonderful tool in your halitosis battling arsenal.

Herbal Remedy – Anise
Anise seeds can be used to create a mouthwash or drink that has been found to be highly effective in battling bad breath. Please note that the seeds should be boiled before use for the highest degree of effectiveness.

Herbal Remedy – Ayurveda
Ayurveda can freshen breath when chewed for a few minutes (found in fennel seeds). This is supported by research done by Dr. Vasant Lad, BA, MS, MA, Director of the Ayurvedic Institute in Albuquerque, New Mexico.

Herbal Remedy – Cardam Om
Cardam Om is known for its antiseptic properties, helping to eradicate bacteria and thus decrease bad breath. You chew on cardam om for a few minutes and then spit them out – do not swallow.

Herbal Remedy – Eucalyptus
Eucalyptus is often used in mouthwashes, however you can simply chew on eucalyptus leaves and experience a brief re-freshening of your breath. Great, natural remedy.

Hydrogen Peroxide
Hydrogen peroxide kills bacteria. Use extreme caution when using this however, you should not use hydrogen peroxide at a concentration of any higher than 1.5% - to achieve this you must mix hydrogen peroxide with water and a pinch of salt.

You also should not swallow hydrogen peroxide, as this can be fatal. Hydrogen peroxide kills bacteria of all kinds – and you need a lot of bacterias to thrive in terms of your health, so only use this extremely carefully and do NOT use excessively.

Parsley
Parsley contains chlorophyll, a substance known to freshen breath. Consumption should occur only when parsley has been prepared, and can serve to help increase your immune system and mental alertness while freshening your breath.

How to prepare parsley: Chop up a bit of parsley, boil it with ground or whole cloves and two cups of water. Strain out leaves and pieces of clove. Use the remaining liquid as a mouthwash.

Peppermint

Peppermint is found in mints, in candies, in gum, in toothpaste, and also in tea. Peppermint tea in particular can be a great tool in battling bad breath.

Paw Paw
Paw paw is a type of fruit which has become known for their cleansing abilities. For a great dessert, cut open some paw paw, remove its seeds, and cut into small pieces. Eating a few of these fruit pieces a day can aid your battle against bad breath considerably.

Tea
In addition to peppermint tea, teas in general have been found to aid in the fight against halitosis. This is thought to be because the polyphenols properties within tea halt bacteria's growth, thus slowing the production of VSC's, and reducing bad breath.

Triple Complex Hali Tonic
This is a 'medicine' advocated by naturopaths for the treatment of bad breath. See below for more information.

Yoghurt
Yoghurt can help in the battle against bad breath, and in the aiding of your oral hygiene health (it has been linked to reductions in decay and disease). However, it should be noted that these effects are held to be in sugarless yoghurts, so watch your labels when selecting one to take home.

Triple Complex Hali Tonic
Native Remedies, an advocating company for

natural remedies, has established this tonic comprised of a variety of natural herbs known to help combat the issue of bad breath.

What it Does
- Helps with gum disease and health issues related to the stomach
- Freshens your breath
- Targets the root causes of halitosis and addresses them by cleansing the body of bacteria

What it Contains
Triple Complex Hali Tonic contains a number of herbs, but the primary ones will be listed here. You should always do your research when considering taking a tonic, you need to know what's going into your body.

- Kalium Phosphate
  This is a biochemical agent which acts in an antiseptic capacity, eliminating bacteria, cleansing your body, and reducing bodily decay. This substance has been known to help not just with halitosis, but also with flatulence.

- Lactose
  It should be noted that the amount of lactose in Hali Tonic is small enough that even individuals who suffer from issues with lactose are able to take it.

- Milk Thistle
  Milk thistle, aka carduus marianus, works to enhance the functioning of the liver. The liver is responsible for filtering in your system, and thus milk thistle helps in the cleansing process but more importantly stimulates your body in the cleansing process of toxic substances (including excessive VSCs).

- Silica
  Warning: Should not be used by people with breast implants, prosthetic limbs, pace makers, pins, or other foreign substances. Its cleansing properties are extreme and harm will come if used by these people.

Also known as silicone dioxide, silica is known for being a practical 'homeopathic surgeon'. Its abilities come in not just in reducing the body of odor, but also in battling gum disease, abscesses, and purifying the body.

- Sweet Fennel
  Sweet fennel, also known as foeniculum vulgare, acts in multiple ways for the body. Its primary use has been as a digestive aid, as it acts as a calming agent on the body, relieving spasming of the organs and thus reducing discomfort.

How it Works
Triple Complex Hali Tonic cleanses the areas of bacteria and works in conjunction with good oral

hygiene habits to not only eliminate your bad breath temporarily, but rather eradicate your halitosis permanently.

Conclusion

Herbs, fruits, and even medicines, are not the only forms of alternative treatment. Naturopathy also encompasses remedies and alternative holistic approaches to wellness, and we will now consider some of those methods in the chapters to come.

Remedies You Can Make at Home

The following are recipes for homemade tools of the trade: mouthwashes, toothpaste, and cleansers. They place emphasis on inexpensive, common, household items, to emphasize the natural ability to combat bad breath issues.

Cleansers
Fruit Cleanser
Lemons and strawberries (used separately) can be used to remove stains from your teeth!

Step 1) Rub lemon rind along stains
Step 2) Rinse

Old Fashioned Powder
Ingredients
- 2 tsp. salt
- 2 Tbsp. dried orange or lemon rind
- 1/4 cup baking soda

Instructions
Step 1) Grind rinds into a powder (can use processer for this)
Step 2) Combine with soda and salt
Step 3) Can be used as a paste or with toothbrush dipping

Lemon Clove Cleanser
Ingredients

- 10 drops of clove oil
- 12 drops of bergamot oil
- 20 drops lemon oil
- Pinch of fine sage
- 1 ounce finely powdered myrrh
- 3 ounces powdered orrisroot
- 1 pound powdered arrowroot

Instructions
Step 1) Combine dry ingredients
Step 2) Add oils drop by drop, mixing thoroughly

This can be used on an as-needed basis

Super Cleanser
Ingredients
- Baking soda
- Few drops of hydrogen peroxide

Instructions
Step 1) Mix ingredients together
Step 2) The resulting paste can be used on your teeth daily and on your gums no more than two times per week.

Toothpastes
The instructions portion of the toothpaste recipes is the same for all of the recipes.
Step 1) Mix the ingredients
Step 2) Store in airtight container

Ben Franklin's Toothpaste
Ingredients
- Ground charcoal
- Honey

Loretta's Toothpaste
Ingredients
- 1/4 tsp. hydrogen peroxide
- 1 tsp. baking soda
- 1 drop peppermint oil

Mint Toothpaste
Ingredients
- 1/3 tsp. salt
- 4 tsp. glycerin
- 6 tsp. baking soda
- 15 drops peppermint or wintergreen

Simple Toothpaste
Ingredients
- Baking soda
- Glycerin
- Peppermint oil
- Salt
- Water

Steps: Mix to a paste wherein the ratio of baking soda to salt is 3 to 1, and glycerin is a maximum of 3 tsp. to 1/4 cup mix.

Tasty Toothpaste Recipe
Ingredients

- 1/4 tsp. spearmint
- 1/4 tsp. peppermint oil
- 1 tsp. ground sage
- 1/4 cup arrowroot
- 1/4 cup powdered orrisroot
- 1/4 cup water

Try this one with cinnamon or cloves instead of peppermint for fun!

Vanilla and Rose Geranium Toothpaste
Ingredients
- 1/2 ounce powdered chalk
- 3 ounces powdered orrisroot
- 4 tsp. tincture of vanilla
- 15 drops of rose geranium oil
- Enough honey that it turns into a paste

Mouthwashes
Baking Soda Mouthwash
Ingredients
- 2 ounces water
- 1/4 tsp. baking soda
- 1 drop tea tree oil
- 1 drop peppermint oil

Instructions
Step 1) Mix the ingredients
Step 2) Use as a mouth wash (yes it's this simple

Rosemary-Mint Mouthwash
Ingredients
- 2 1/2 cups water (distilled or mineral only)

- 1 tsp. anise seeds
- 1 tsp. fresh mint
- 1 tsp. rosemary leaves

Instructions

Step 1) Boil the water, combining the ingredients in the heated pot.

Step 2) Allow to cool, removing from the heated element

Step 3) Strain the liquid into a container (the goal being to remove leaves)

Step 4) Use as a mouthwash

Spearmint Mouthwash

Ingredients
- 1 tsp. aloe vera
- 4 tsp. liquid glycerin
- 6 ounces of water
- 2 ounces of vodka
- 10-15 drops Spearmint essential oil

Instructions

Step 1) Boil the vodka and water together

Step 2) Add in the aloe vera and the glycerin

Step 3) Cool

Step 4) Add in spearmint

Step 5) Pour into container, shake, and use as mouthwash

Simplest Mouthwash Ever

Ingredients
- 8 ounces of warm water
- 1 tsp. salt

Instructions
Gargle, swish around your mouth, and rinse.

Other Alternative Treatments

Halitosis can be treated in a variety of ways, this chapter overviews a few of the non-recipe related ones.

Aromatherapy
Victoria Edwards, respected aromatherapist in Fair Oaks, California has said that placing just a drop of peppermint oil on the tongue can be enough to make a huge difference.

Food Therapy
Dr. Delson Haas, MD, director of the Preventive Medical Center of Marin in San Rafael, California, says that bad breath has been directly linked to an increase in yeast and dairy substances. Dr. Haas thus recommends limiting alcohol, vinegar, and sugar intake and increasing your intake of fruits and vegetables.

Bad breath can be caused from many things, as we now know, some of these things can be solved with changes in diet. This is because gum disease and issues within the body have both been implicated as potential causes of bad breath.

So, what are the other dietary recommendations?
- Eat more of yogurt and other acidophilus rich foods
- Eat more of plaque fighting foods (Carrots, celery, cheese, peanuts)
- Eat more fruits and vegetables (especially

parsley!)
- Eat fiber rich foods

Herbal Therapy
See the above chapter on treatments for more information, but numerous researchers recommend this, particularly the chewing of seeds, to fight bad breath.

Homeopathy
Homeopaths typically recommend an additional intake of Mercurius, generally 30X dose 3-4 times a day, according to Richard D. Fischer, D.D.S in Annandale Virginia, and President of the International Academy of Oral Medicine and Toxicology.

Hydrotherapy
See the above chapter on the importance of remaining hydrated. Dr. Agatha Thrash, MD of Seale Alabama, recommends mixing in anise, caraway, or cinnamon to add to your benefits of water drinking.

Reflexology
The reflexologist can hit certain parts of the body that can stimulate the cleansing of the body, which helps your battle against halitosis. Dwight Byers, reflexologist from St Petersburg, Florida emphasizes the importance of hitting the points for the stomach, liver, and intestines. This means focusing on foot massage along the sides of your feet and bottoms of your toes.

Yoga

Dr. Stephen A. Nezezon, yoga teacher at the Himalayan International Institute of Yoga Science and Philosophy in Hosedale, Pennsylvania states that the head-to-knee pose may be a particularly critical yogic technique that may improve the functioning of the body and thus battle halitosis.

Preventing Halitosis from Returning

Treating halitosis is important, but it's also critical to assure it doesn't get the power to come back once banished. By working with these simple steps, you will ensure that you are taking care of your mouth, and thus make it significantly more difficult for halitosis to return.

The Methods:
- Use the right tools
  - ☐ Select your toothbrush and toothpaste carefully, select the right mouthwash, set yourself up for success
- Always work to keep your oral hygiene habits up
  - ☐ Brush your teeth every day
  - ☐ Floss
  - ☐ Use mouthwash
  - ☐ Review earlier chapters as necessary for guidelines on this
- Regularly consult with a dental professional to catch oral health issues before they cause bigger problems

Tips to Ensure your Success
We all know how to brush our teeth by now hopefully, but the following are tips collected from the ADA and elsewhere, that should act as additional helpful hints on how to brush properly. Taking care of your mouth is important, take it seriously.

Brushing Tips
Step 1) Hold your toothbrush against your teeth at a 45 degree angle.

Step 2) Gently brush back and forth in short strokes, making sure you clean your teeth, your tongue, your cheeks and your lips.

Step 3) Turn the brush to a 90 degree angle and brush your upper and lower teeth

How to Clean your Tongue
Step 1) Use an antibacterial mouthwash to soak your toothbrush for a few seconds

Step 2) Reach back within your mouth, using the toothbrush to reach as far as you can on your tongue without gagging, and gently clean

Step 3) Rinse the toothbrush well and repeat as necessary

Flossing Tips
Step 1) Use 15 inches of strong floss, winding around the middle finger on one hand and another finger on the other hand.

Step 2) Hold the floss tightly between your fingers

Step 3) Gently go back and forth with the floss between each of your teeth (TIP: If you find your floss is snapping, you are not being gentle enough)

Step 4) Repeat this process for between each of your teeth

Mouthwash Tips
- Select a mouthwash carefully
- Follow the instructions of your chosen mouthwash!

Dos and Don'ts with Oral Health

Promoting your oral health is about a lot more than making sure you're brushing. It's about making sure you're flossing too, you're brushing right, and more. Cleaning your teeth is about more than just battling halitosis, it's also about maintaining good oral health. If you ignore the tips provided in this guide, you run the serious risk of cavities, gum disease, and potentially even more serious health consequences.

A key example of the importance of oral health is illustrated in the effects of plaque. Plaque is a substance that builds up from groups of bacteria that stick to your teeth. If left alone, plaque will attack your gums, increasing their tenderness and causing them to potentially bleed. If you ignore this symptom, gum disease kicks in and the gums begin to try to withdraw from the teeth. This is where you get into much more serious infections, and possibly even tooth loss.

The following is a list of helpful Do's and Do Not's... which again should act as a guide to help you prevent the return of halitosis.

DO

- Brush at least once a day, hopefully 2-3 times for a few minutes at a time
- Floss
- Hydrate
- Consider how your diet may be impacting your breath and oral health
- Chew sugar free gum
- Regularly consult with a dental professional
- Soak your dentures in antiseptic solution unless otherwise instructed

DON'T

- Ignore your gums, your tongue, or flossing needs
- Ignore oral health issues
- Be too hard on your mouth, this will lead to bleeding and pain, not recovery and prevention
- Use mouthwash with children
- Skip dental appointments

Conclusions

You've reached the end! You now understand bad breath, the causes behind it, and your treatment options. Always remember you can always do more research, or consult with the American Dental Association, if you're still having questions.

Don't forget to follow through with the things you've learned here. Review chapters as necessary. Set cell phone reminders to brush multiple times per day. Make sure you're using the right tools for you.

Most importantly? Seek help. You know that you're not alone in this struggle. No one is. This is the struggle of millions of people around the world, and although you may be tempted to feel alone – don't give in.

On the flip side of this, make sure if you know someone who is struggling with bad breath, you find a way to get this information to them. It could be as easy as discussing the book or leaving it around on your computer. The point is, it's much needed for many people, and getting people help doesn't have to be humiliating.

Call a Dentist (or Doctor) if. . .
- If pain accompanies your halitosis

- If you are bleeding or losing teeth

- If you have a fever

>> <u>Sign Up for our Exclusive Health Newsletter TODAY!</u> <<
www.naturesnaturalhealth.com/join/

www.ingramcontent.com/pod-product-compliance
Lightning Source LLC
Chambersburg PA
CBHW070339290526
45791CB00003B/1400